The Ultimate Runner's Diet

How to Fuel Your Body for Peak Running Performance

J. M. Parker

ISBN-13: 978-1479300143

ISBN-10: 1479300144

Disclaimer

This book is copyrighted with all rights reserved. No part of this book may be used in any form, physical or electronic, without express permission from the author.

The author does not assume any liability for the use or misuse of information contained herein. The information contained within this guide is for educational purposes and is offered as-is. The author does not assume any responsibility for the accuracy or misuse of any information contained herein.

While every attempt has been made to provide information that is both accurate and proven effective, the author and publisher make no guarantees that the information presented herein will benefit everyone in every situation. Everyone's situation is unique. The author assumes no liabilities for any use, misuse, injury or misconduct as a result of information within this book. As with all things that have to do with your body, if in doubt consult with your health care practitioner.

Table of Contents

About the Author

The author is a twelve year Army veteran who used to train soldiers to remain in compliance with Army height and weight standards in order to help them keep their careers. She has worked with many soldiers to complete the Army Birthday Annual Ten-Miler, and to get them down to a healthy height and weight. She is also certified to work with pregnant and post-partum women to safely maintain their fitness during pregnancy and to bounce back after child birth.

Post Army, the author still leads an active lifestyle and is pursuing a physical training certification and training for a local marathon. Diet being a major contributor to peak performance in running and in life.

Also by J. M. Parker

The Ultimate Running Guide: How To Train For a 5K, 10K, Half-Marathon or Full Marathon (Kindle edition)

The Ultimate Running Guide (Paperback edition)

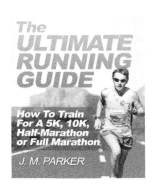

Intro To Your Best Running Diet Ever

Do you like to run? You should! Running is an outstanding activity that increases your cardio respiratory capacity, helps you maintain or lose weight and helps prevent heart disease and certain cancers. Running can be aerobic or anaerobic, meaning you can perform for a long time at a sustained pace (aerobic), or you can do it in very fast, short bursts (anaerobic). Both zones have benefits. Aerobic exercise is considered the fat burning zone, because your body uses fat stores to fuel itself for the workout. Anaerobic is excellent for strengthening your heart and torching hundreds of calories in a short amount of time.

Running also gives you that awesome, "runner's high." Sure, it's a cliché, but the endorphin spike experienced from a good running work out is almost thrilling. It's also a great social activity. You can get together with a bunch of friends and train for running events together. Or if you prefer, it's a great solitary activity. Fewer things clear your head like running for miles while the world passes you by.

Running is essentially useless though, if the runner isn't properly fueled for performance. Every athlete should follow a diet plan specific to his or her training. Body builders should consume more protein. Gymnasts need more calcium. If you are reading this, you're probably a runner. You need more carbohydrates. The great thing about being a runner is, you're allowed more carbohydrates than many athletes, and even more so than those who live an unmotivated, sedentary lifestyle.

Over the years carbs have been demonized by nutritionists and other professionals. They have been accused of being empty calories and as being stored as fat if they aren't burned soon enough. You don't need to worry about this as much if you're a runner. They'll burn right off, if you do it right. Repeat after me: Carbohydrates are your friends.

Be aware though, you can't be buddies with every carbohydrate you meet. Your carbohydrates should come primarily from complex sources, such as whole grain bread, rice and flour. Whole grains deliver a variety of nutrients such as magnesium and selenium and they are more difficult for your body to metabolize, making you feel full longer. Simple carbs are found in foods such as fruits, bleached flour and white rice. The simple carbohydrates in fruits are fine, because they deliver nutritional benefits, but products containing bleached flour are nutrient-free calorie bombs.

Many products that are made with white flour or white rice are enriched with vitamins and minerals. So what's the point of that? They strip everything out, then add the stuff back in. Does that even sound like its good for you? I didn't think so. At all times possible, food is best consumed close to its original form. This means, unbleached, unrefined, un-enriched and recognizable as what they were before they hit the stores.

But enough about carbs. I think we've cleared that up. You need more than sugars to keep you in tip-top running form.

Also important are protein, calcium and healthy fats, such as those found in avocados, salmon, and nuts. The majority of your energy will come from carbohydrates, but protein aids in recovery and muscle building, calcium keeps your bones strong so they can support your body during exercise, and healthy fats help you absorb vitamins and minerals more efficiently.

A long distance runner, who clocks more than 20 miles each week should get about sixty percent of their calories from complex carbohydrate sources, about thirty percent should come from protein sources, and the rest should come from fat.

So now I bet you think you have all the answers don't you? You think you can just throw your sneakers on and get going. Think again. You need a plan of action before you set out on your running adventures. What are you going to eat before a run? What type of recovery drink (if any) do you plan to consume after? Should you use supplements? If you don't know the answers to these questions, then you are not ready in the diet department of your running regime. That's ok though. We are here to get you ready. Intrigued? Put down the doughnuts and read on.

Before Your Run

Many athletes, runners included, make the mistake of exercising on an empty stomach. When you run, especially when you run long distances, you are using a LOT of energy. Food gives you energy, so it's vital to eat before you hit the track (or hills, or shoulder of the road). No one is telling you to run to your local greasy spoon and stuff yourself with a bacon cheeseburger and other fatty, salty nonsense. We are just letting you know you need to eat prior to your workout, so that you aren't totally fatigued by the end of it.

Remember when we spoke of the different types of carbs? This is one of those instances in which you will want to go for simple carbs. Put the cookies down!! We didn't say refined carbohydrates, we said simple, and we were referring to the simple carbs found in fruits such as apples, bananas, and melon. Not only will these foods fuel you for your workout, but they also have high water content, helping to keep you hydrated. Hydration is essential to your success as well. More about that later.

The following is four weeks worth of ideas for your pre-run snacks. Bear in mind, you should take two days out of the week for recovery, so there will only be five items for each week.

Week 1

Monday: Banana with ½ cup non-fat plain yogurt (Greek is best, but not essential) Bananas are high in potassium, which helps prevent those annoying muscle spasms during your run. Yogurt delivers an excellent mix of carbs and protein.

Tuesday: Apple with 1TBS almond or peanut butter. High in both carbs and water, apples are one of the best pre-run foods. Peanut and almond butters contain healthy fats and protein.

Wednesday: Melon slices with ½ cup non-fat cottage cheese. Melon is high on the list of carbohydrate rich fruits. Like yogurt, cottage cheese provides a nice balance of protein and carbs.

Thursday: Pineapple slices and 1 hardboiled egg. Pineapple is full of antioxidants that fight free-radicals, which cause damage to your cells and annoyances such as pre-mature aging and cancer. Everyone knows how good eggs are for you. Low in calories and high in protein, they are quite possibly the gold standard of healthy eating. Yes, you can eat the yolk.

Saturday: Figs with 1 cup of almond milk. Figs taste great and are rich in carbs. Almond milk provides the same amount of protein as cow's milk, but for half the calories. It's a great option if you are trying to lose weight, or if you're lactose intolerant and don't like soy milk.

Week 2

Monday: Half a mango and 1 slice turkey bacon. Mangos are typically very big, which is why we suggest just half. Turkey bacon is low in fat, and high in protein, but it also has a very high sodium content, so we recommend no more than one slice.

Tuesday: Two tangerines and a slice of low-fat cheese. Tangerines are very small, so it's ok to have two of them. They are water-dense and provide about 9 grams of carbohydrates. Just like the other dairy products we keep talking about cheese is great for a good balance of carbs and protein.

Wednesday: 20 grapes and 1 cup almond milk. Grapes are excellent for hydration and carbohydrates. Individually, they don't deliver much, since they are so small, but 20 of them will give you about 18 grams of carbohydrates.

Thursday: 1 Orange and 10 cashews. A single orange provides about 15 grams of carbohydrates. Cashews are excellent if you like salty foods. While they are higher in fat than we'd normally recommend prior to a workout, the 9 grams of carbs make them worth it.

Saturday: Cantaloupe slices and 5 almonds. Of course the cantaloupe is high in carbohydrates, and water, just like the rest of the fruits we have recommended. Almonds are similar to cashews in fat content, but 95 grams of almonds will give you a whopping 20 grams of carbs.

Week 3

Monday: 20 Cherries and a small handful of almonds. Cherries have a good water content and plenty of carbohydrates. The almonds help offset the tangy sweetness of the cherries and provide you with some protein and omega-3 fatty acids.

Tuesday: Mango chunks and whole wheat toast with peanut butter. Mango is full of water, carbs and electrolytes. The wheat bread gives an extra boost of carbohydrates while the peanut butter delivers muscle repairing protein.

Wednesday: Half a grapefruit with a cup of green tea and a small handful of cashews. Grapefruit is very water and carbohydrate dense. Green tea contains antioxidants and is said to increase metabolism. The cashews will help your muscles recover with protein.

Thursday: Watermelon slices and whole wheat bagel with fat free cream cheese and one cup of coconut water. The watermelon, as its name suggests provides tons of water. The bagel and cream cheese combo is the perfect protein and carbohydrate mix. The coconut water is full of electrolytes, which you can front-load before your run.

Saturday: Low fat/low sugar granola with melon slices and green tea. Get your carb fix from the granola, and water from the melon. The green tea supplies energy (if you need the caffeine boost) and antioxidants.

Week 4

Monday: Strawberries, raspberries and blackberries with almond slivers and a cup of almond milk. Berries are full of flavor, water and antioxidants, while almonds and almond milk deliver the protein needed to aid in muscle recovery.

Tuesday: One pear, one apple and whole wheat toast with peanut butter. Apples and pears are full of fiber, carbs and water. Get even more carbohydrates from the toast and protein from the peanut butter.

Wednesday: Orange slices and string cheese with coconut water. Get much needed hydration from the oranges and coconut water and some protein from the string cheese. This combo is great for those who like to eat light before working out.

Thursday: Peach slices and cashews with almond milk. Peaches have a good amount of fiber, but they don't feel "heavy" so they are ideal prior to running. They also have a high water content. Get your protein fill from the cashews and almond milk.

Saturday: Kiwi slices and whole wheat toast with sugar free jam. Kiwi is packed full of water and tastes amazing. The whole wheat toast and jam deliver plenty of carbohydrates to fuel your run. This is a good choice if you can't stomach protein prior to your run.

These guidelines are not the end all, be all of your pre-run snacking. You may need to cut the protein sources in these snacks, or save them for post workout. You may need to do the same with dairy. You may need to up the amount of food you eat before your run, or reduce it depending on your running regime. Experiment and see which formula works best for you. So long as you toss those fatty cakes out the window and eat right. Eat right and you will BE right.

The magic formula is different for everyone, so if one of your running buddies can tolerate protein and dairy before a run, but it doesn't work for you, don't fret. So long as your nutritional needs are met throughout the day, you'll be just fine.

After a Run

After you've completed a run, it's time to fuel your body for recovery. Runners use nearly their entire bodies when they run, and your muscles will need some help in repairing themselves after such an intense ordeal.

This is where the protein is especially important. You still need carbs after a run to replenish the energy you've expended. But protein is your muscles' building blocks, so this is when you'll really want to focus on it.

Every meal on our four-week plan for before a run will work for after a run as well. If you skipped the protein pre-run, it's a good idea to eat it after the run (with another carbohydrate source). However, you can do better than just those two weeks worth of snacks. You don't want to get bored, because boredom is what makes you reach for those fatty cakes.

Since we care about you and want to make sure you keep those fatty cakes away, we've come up with four weeks worth of post-run meals as well. Put the doughnuts down and read on.

Week 1

Monday: Greek Yogurt with sliced strawberries, almond slivers and blueberries. Greek yogurt has more protein than regular yogurt, so it's a better post-run choice. Blueberries and strawberries give the yogurt flavor and give your body antioxidants and vitamin C, to keep you healthy and keep you on that track.

Tuesday: Chocolate Milk and cashews. Yes, you read that right. You can have chocolate milk, so long as you use a low sugar chocolate mix. Milk has the perfect ratio of carbohydrates and proteins, making it an excellent recovery drink after a long run. This is an especially good recovery formula for females, who tend to lack calcium. For a low sugar drink, mix 1 tablespoon of unsweetened coco powder into an 8 ounce glass of milk. Add 1.5 teaspoons of vanilla extract, and 1 teaspoon of Stevia, a plant based sugar substitute. Cashews provide a little more protein, and help you feel full.

Wednesday: Half of a whole grain bagel with two tablespoons of low fat cream cheese. The bagel will help replenish your carbs, and the cream cheese gives you a good dose of protein, calcium and yes, carbohydrates. Have a side of fruit if you'd like something more substantial.

Thursday: Two hard boiled eggs and an orange. Eggs are one of the best sources of lean protein available. Even better? They are one of the few items in your grocery store that's still reasonably priced. The orange delivers some carbohydrates, and has a lot of water in it, helping to hydrate you.

Saturday: 1 slice of whole grain toast with almond butter and a cup of almond milk, watermelon slices (You can make it chocolate like Tuesday, if you'd like). The almond milk is a tasty, healthy alternative to cow's milk. Almond butter tastes really fresh and has less sugar than peanut butter. Watermelon is another water and carbohydrate rich fruit that helps to replace expended carbohydrates and water.

Week 2

Monday: 1 Cup coconut water, Greek yogurt with raspberries and a drizzle of honey. Coconut water is an outstanding source of potassium, helping to prevent muscle spasms. It helps hydrate you and stave off the boredom of water. As mentioned, Greek yogurt has more protein than regular yogurt, to aid in muscle recovery. Raspberries are a tasty source of antioxidants and vitamin C, to keep you race ready! Honey is a healthy substitute for sugar and helps tame the tang of plain Greek yogurt.

Tuesday: Whole grain cereal (oatmeal and whole grain Cream of Wheat are excellent choices) topped with berries of your choice and low fat milk. This well rounded meal has everything you need for a speedy recovery, all in one bowl. The cereal and berries have the carbs and slow burn fiber to keep you energized until lunch time. The milk, of course gives that great balance of protein and carbohydrates.

Wednesday: Whole wheat tortilla with 2 scrambled egg whites, low fat cheese (feta is really good), diced tomatoes and spinach. Get your whole grains from the tortilla, vitamins from the spinach and tomatoes and protein and extra carbs from the cheese.

Thursday: Whole grain, sugar free waffles, sugar free syrup, hard-boiled egg and melon balls. Whole grain waffles are a healthy take on the breakfast favorite, and more satisfying than those made with bleached flour. The egg gives you your protein source and the melons help you hydrate.

Saturday: Turkey sausage with whole grain toast and two eggs scrambled with diced bell peppers, tomatoes and low fat cheddar cheese. If you're a meat lover, but don't love the effects of animal fat, turkey sausage is a great way to get your fix without the fat. This meal gives you lots of protein for muscle recovery at the end of your run week, and the additions to the eggs sneak in some extra nutrients.

Week 3

Monday: Whole wheat, sugar free pancakes topped with strawberries, blackberries and blueberries with two hardboiled eggs and coconut water. Replenish your carbohydrates with the pancakes and your water and electrolytes with the fruit and coconut water. The eggs provide enough protein to aid in the repair of your torn muscles.

Tuesday: Whole wheat tortilla filled with egg whites, low-fat turkey sausage, spinach and tomatoes with a side of your choice of fruit. This filling meal is great for runners who feel totally famished after a workout. The eggs and turkey sausage deliver tons of protein, which fills you up and helps your muscles out. The fruit serves to replace some of your water and carbohydrates that were lost during your run.

Wednesday: Egg white omelet filled with feta cheese, spinach, diced tomatoes and mushrooms. Spinach is the one veggie that works in several different breakfast meals and it's full of iron and other essential nutrients. Egg whites are outstanding sources of low fat, low calorie protein sources. Tomatoes provide lycopene, which is thought to prevent certain cancers, and water. Mushrooms are full of nutritional benefits, including vitamin D and potassium.

Thursday: Whole wheat French toast slice topped with strawberries and blueberries with a slice of turkey bacon. Coat your bread slices with egg whites and fry it in a fat-free pan spray to keep this tasty treat low calorie. Get a carbohydrate refill from the fruit and bread and get your protein from the turkey bacon.

Saturday: Low fat/low sugar granola with plain Greek yogurt, honey, berries and almonds. Either mix it all up and enjoy, or layer it parfait style. The granola and berries will give you your carbohydrate refill while the yogurt and almonds provide much needed protein. The honey is an excellent low calorie sweetener.

Week 4

Monday: 2 hard-boiled eggs with apple slices and peanut butter and one cup of coconut water. This protein rich meal has everything you need to recover from a distance run or a short/fast run. The eggs and peanut butter are chock-full of protein while the apple slices replace some of your lost carbohydrates. Coconut water is a great tasting electrolyte-rich option.

Tuesday: egg whites scrambled with feta cheese, diced tomatoes and spinach. Serve with a side of whole grain toast and a banana. The omelet is overflowing with protein and the rich nutritional benefits of tomatoes and spinach. Get your carb fix from the toast and banana. The added bonus? The banana also delivers potassium, which helps prevent muscle spasms.

Wednesday: Bagel breakfast sandwich: Toast a whole wheat bagel and spread some mustard on it. Fry an egg in fat free pan spray until the yolk is cooked through. Place the egg, a turkey sausage patty and a tomato slice in between. You can make your eggs sunny-side up or over-easy, but that will make for a messy sandwich. Serve with a side of your choice of fruit. This meal has tons of protein and is low in fat and calories. Replace your carbohydrates and water with the fruit and the bagel. You can also make these sandwiches ahead of time so you're ready for those hectic mornings when you need a grab n' go option.

Thursday: Fat free cottage cheese with peach slices and a side of whole wheat toast with almond butter. The cottage cheese and almond butter provide your protein while the peaches and toast replenish your carbohydrates. For an additional nutrition boost, drink some antioxidant rich green tea.

Saturday: Breakfast B.L.T. Toast some whole wheat bread. Spread some low fat butter substitute or fat free mayo on the bread. Place a slice of turkey bacon, a tomato slice and a slice of romaine lettuce between your bread slices. Enjoy with a side of Greek yogurt topped with berries. This low fat version of a classic B.L.T. has all the components of an excellent post-run meal: protein, carbohydrates and water.

All of the post run meals are recommended under the assumption that you run in the morning. If you're an evening runner, these meals will still work, but if you're the type that wants "breakfast" foods at "breakfast" you may need to adjust. Replace eggs with lean fish, chicken or turkey, or lean cuts of red meat. Replace the fruits with veggies. Do whatever you need to do to modify the meal to meet your needs.

As with the "before you run" meals, you can add or subtract to these recommendations as you see fit to meet your specific needs for top performance. Just leave the fatty cakes alone and fuel your body the right way.

Daily Diet

The meals we gave for Before and After a run are just snacks, although, with some extra fruit added to the "after" portions they could serve as breakfast, if you'd prefer. Of course, a snack before a run and one after isn't enough to get you through the day. You still have to go to work, clean your house, run errands, and tend to all those other pesky, energy draining activities. The four week plan that follows gives you meal and snack options to keep your energy up and your waistline down throughout the day.

Week 1

Monday

Breakfast
-Two hard-boiled eggs (you can eat the yolk)
-Smoothie containing 1 banana, 4 strawberries, 10 blackberries, a half a cup of Greek yogurt, either plain or vanilla, a few spinach leaves and ice. (don't worry about the spinach, you won't taste it, but you WILL reap the benefits of it.) Grind it all up and enjoy. Use honey or agave nectar to sweeten it. Also, you can use frozen fruit and skip the ice to save time.
-Granola bar (make sure it's low sugar, organic is best)
Lunch

-Salad with baby spinach leaves or romaine lettuce, tomatoes, kidney beans, sunflower seeds, broccoli florets and grilled chicken strips.

-Use low fat dressing, or Balsamic vinegar and extra virgin olive oil. Feel free to add more veggies to this if you'd like

Dinner

-Grilled fish (salmon, tilapia, halibut, tuna fish, etc.)

-Steamed mixed vegetables

-Roasted red potatoes with rosemary and cherry tomatoes.

Tuesday

Breakfast

-Whole grain bagel with one Laughing Cow or Weight Watchers cheese wedge.

-One half grapefruit, sweetened with Stevia

-1 strip of turkey bacon

Lunch

-Turkey breast sandwich on whole grain bread with lettuce and tomatoes

-Garden salad or minestrone soup

-Low-fat yogurt

Dinner
-Grilled chicken breast
-Steamed asparagus
-Brown Rice

Wednesday

Breakfast
-Greek yogurt with honey and granola
-Skim milk latte
-Cup of sliced melon
Lunch
-Veggie burger on whole grain bun with lettuce and tomatoes
-Steamed mixed veggies
-Frozen baked French fries
Dinner
-3 oz lean steak
-Summer squash
-Baked Sweet potato

Thursday

Breakfast
-Whole grain cereal (Kashi and Special K make excellent ones) with skim milk
-Orange slices
-Whole grain toast with peanut butter
Lunch

-Whole grain pita with chicken breast, plain Greek yogurt, tomatoes and olives
-Garden salad
Dinner
-Whole grain spaghetti with marinara sauce and ground turkey meat balls
-Bruschetta with whole grain bread

Friday

Breakfast
-Oatmeal with walnuts, milk honey and cinnamon
-Apple
Lunch
-Tomato soup with Triscuits
-Baby carrots and fat free cream cheese
Dinner
-Chicken fajitas with fat free sour cream on whole grain tortillas

Saturday

Breakfast
-Egg White omelets with low fat cheddar cheese, diced green peppers, tomatoes and low-fat ham
-Bowl of mixed fruits
Lunch
-Grilled Chicken salad
- Your choice of low fat soup
Dinner
-Roasted pork loin

-Boiled artichokes
-Roasted russet potatoes

Sunday

Breakfast
-Whole grain waffles with sugar free syrup
-Strawberry and blackberry parfait
Lunch
-Spaghetti squash with marinara sauce
-Grilled chicken breast
Dinner
-Grilled fish
-Steamed broccoli
-Baked russet potatoes

Week 2

Monday

Breakfast
-1 Cup shredded whole wheat cereal (sugar free) topped with sliced strawberries, raspberries and bananas. Use low fat or almond milk
-1 Slice of whole grain toast with almond butter
Lunch
-Low-sodium vegetable soup with a whole grain bread roll
- Celery stalks with low-fat cream cheese
Dinner
-Turkey Burgers on whole grain buns, with baked sweet potato fries and a veggie of your choice

Tuesday

Breakfast
-Two slices of whole grain French toast. Use fat-free non-stick spray to fry the bread. Top with berries or sugar free syrup.
-Scramble the left-over egg coating and eat with the French toast

Lunch
-Chili made with lean ground turkey
-Side salad with baby spinach leaves, cherry tomatoes, diced cucumbers, shredded carrots and snap-peas

Dinner
-3oz baked salmon fillet with
-Baked sweet potato
-Baked squash of your choice

Wednesday

Breakfast
-Non-fat yogurt with mixed berries and low sugar granola
-Whole wheat toast

Lunch
-Grilled chicken breast on a whole grain bun
-Baked French fries
-Peas and carrots

Dinner

Chicken parmesan. Coat chicken with whole-wheat breadcrumbs and bake until chicken is cooked through. Top with marinara sauce and fresh grated parmesan cheese. Serve with salad and whole grain bread.

Thursday

Breakfast
-Oatmeal topped with cinnamon, diced apples and almond slivers
-Mangos and kiwis
Lunch
-Whole wheat pita filled with grilled chicken, hummus, tomatoes, artichoke hearts, olives and cucumbers
Dinner
-Baked pork-chops seasoned with garlic and lemon pepper
-Brown rice
-Mixed veggies

Friday

Breakfast
-Whole wheat pancakes topped with strawberries and low fat whipped topping
Lunch
-Chicken tacos on whole wheat tortillas with guacamole, tomatoes, cilantro and low fat cheese
Dinner
-Oven roasted chicken or store bought rotisserie chicken. Eat the white meat

-Baked potatoes
-Corn

Saturday

Breakfast
-Whole grain Cream of Wheat topped with honey and cinnamon
-Non-fat yogurt with mixed berries
Lunch
-Grilled chicken salad
-Whole grain dinner roll
Dinner
-Grilled shrimp kabobs. Put jumbo shrimp, pineapple chunks, onions and mango chunks on skewers and grill outside or broil in the oven until shrimp is cooked through
-Corn on the cob
-Steamed snap peas

Sunday

Breakfast
-Whole wheat toaster waffles with sugar free syrup
-Orange slices
-Apple slices
-Hard boiled egg
Lunch
-Turkey Sandwich on Rye bread
-Low Sodium vegetable soup
Dinner

-Turkey meatloaf (1lb lean ground turkey, a packet of meatloaf seasoning, 1 small can of tomatoes sauce, ½ cup of oatmeal. Form ingredients into a loaf and bake at 400 degrees for about 30 minutes, or until cooked through)
-Mashed potatoes. Use vegetable stock and low-fat butter to mash.
-Steamed green beans

Week 3

Monday

Breakfast
-Turkey sausage and egg breakfast sandwich
-Fresh fruit
-Honey-drizzled Greek yogurt
Lunch
-Minestrone soup with a whole grain bread roll
-Side salad
Dinner
-Fish wraps (use whole grain tortillas) with mango and pineapple salsa
-Brown rice

Tuesday

Breakfast
-Fruit and yogurt parfait
-Two hardboiled eggs
Lunch
-Grilled chicken breast sandwich and a

-Salad with romaine lettuce, tomatoes, cucumbers sunflower seeds and whatever other greens you'd like to add.

Dinner

-Steamed pork chops with tomato sauce. Place some boneless pork chops in a sauce pan with about an inch of water. Turn heat to medium and cover until chops are cooked through. Pour a can of tomato sauce in the pan and season with garlic, onion, seasoned salt and sofrito. Sofrito is a Spanish cooking base made with cilantro, garlic, onion and green bell peppers. You can buy it or make it. Place chops with sauce over a bed of brown rice.

-Grilled zucchini

Wednesday

Breakfast

-Baked plantain with mango chunks

-Egg white omelet filled with low fat mozzarella cheese, mushrooms, diced tomatoes and spinach.

Plantains are the super-sized version of bananas. They have tons of potassium and carbohydrates. The mango chunks taste good with the plantains and have a high water content. The omelet has tons of protein from the egg whites and mozzarella and the spinach, tomatoes and mushrooms offer tons of nutrients that do everything from prevent cancer to boosting the immune system.

Lunch

-Spaghetti squash spaghetti. Bake some spaghetti squash and top with marinara sauce, grilled chicken slices and fresh grated parmesan cheese
-Side salad
Dinner
-Roasted pork loin
-Peas and carrots
-Whole grain couscous

Thursday

Breakfast
-Oatmeal topped with cinnamon, berries and honey
-Two hard boiled eggs
Lunch
 -Chicken fajita wrap. Place grilled chicken strips, fat free refried beans, salsa, and tomatoes on a whole grain tortilla. Enjoy with a side of Spanish-style brown rice.
Dinner
-Grilled salmon fillet topped with diced mango, pineapple and yellow bell peppers
-zucchini and summer squash fried in olive oil and seasoned with garlic and onion powder

Friday

Breakfast
-Whole wheat French toast topped with sugar free syrup
-Turkey sausage
-Melon balls
Lunch

-Grilled chicken salad with a mix of baby spinach and romaine leave
-Your choice of greens
-If you need something more filling have some fruit on the side.

Dinner
- Lean grilled steak with
-Steamed green beans
-Red potatoes roasted with olive oil, rosemary and cherry tomatoes

Saturday

Breakfast
-Whole wheat bagel with fat free cream cheese
-Two hard boiled eggs
-Peach slices

Lunch
-Grilled turkey sandwich on rye
-Low fat veggie soup

Dinner
-Grilled shrimp salad
-Brown rice pilaf

Sunday

Breakfast
-Whole wheat pancakes topped with non-dairy whipped topping, strawberries and blueberries
-Turkey sausage

Lunch

-Turkey bacon B.L.T.
-Pop-chips or baked sweet potato chips
Dinner
-Grilled chicken with
-Baked sweet potatoes
-Steamed carrots

Week 4

Monday

Breakfast
-Whole grain cereal with almond milk and berries
-Two hardboiled eggs
Lunch
-Turkey burger on a whole grain bun
-Baked potato
-Side salad
Dinner
-Roast pork loin
-Brown rice
-Steamed green beans

Tuesday

Breakfast
-Egg whites scrambled with crumbled turkey sausage and
diced tomatoes
-Side of melon balls

Lunch

-Grilled eggplant
-Grilled chicken sandwich on whole grain bread
-C sticks and hummus
Dinner
-Steak tacos on low fat shells, tomatoes, refried beans, low fat Monterrey jack cheese and salsa.

Wednesday

Breakfast
-Greek yogurt mixed with low fat, whole grain cereal
-Turkey bacon
Lunch
-Low fat chicken soup
-Side salad
-Whole wheat roll
Dinner
-Roasted turkey roll with mashed potatoes (use vegetable stock to mash them)
-Grilled asparagus

Thursday

Breakfast
-Whole grain Cream of Wheat topped with blackberries and honey
-Two hard boiled eggs
Lunch
-Vegetarian hot dogs on whole grain buns
-Baked sweet potato fries
-Kale Chips

Dinner
-Flatbread pizza. Top whole grain flat bread with pizza sauce, low fat mozzarella cheese, tomatoes, feta cheese, olives and Greek peppers. Bake until crust is cooked through.

Friday

Breakfast
-Two baked apples
-Oatmeal topped with honey and cinnamon
-Turkey sausage patty
Lunch
-Black bean burger (You can buy the black bean burgers in most grocery stores)
-Side salad
-Baked frozen fries
Dinner
-Lean steak with
-Baked spaghetti squash
-Red beans and brown rice

Saturday

Breakfast
-Cottage cheese and peaches
-Whole grain toast and almond butter and a side of
-Melon slices
Lunch
-Minestrone soup
-Side salad

Dinner
-Roast chicken breast with
-Baked potato and
-Steamed green beans

Sunday

Breakfast
-Turkey bacon and egg breakfast sandwich
-Peach slices
-Melon balls
Lunch
-Grilled chicken breast
-Whole grain pasta salad
Dinner
-Baked salmon patties (you can use the canned salmon for easier forming)
-Grilled eggplant
-Steamed artichokes

Snacks

-Nuts, especially almonds, cashews and walnuts
-Yogurt
-Low sugar granola
-Skim milk lattes
-Veggies and hummus
-Vegetable chips
-Dried fruit (check sugar content)
-Your choice of fruits and veggies

Dessert Options

-Strawberry shortcake, but use fat free angel food cake
instead of short cake and use fat free whipped topping
-Fruit and yogurt parfait
-Frozen yogurt milk shakes
-Chocolate covered strawberries (in moderation)

The meals and snacks given are such a small portion of the countless options you have that meet both health *and* taste needs. Try your own creations, following our guidelines, or get on the web and search for healthy recipes. There are a million and one ways to properly fuel your body for performance. You don't need deep fried, greasy slop or sugar laden fatty cakes to enjoy the taste of your food.

Dining Out

Here's where sticking to your rules may become difficult. As much as possible, you should eat in to save money *and* calories. However, it's hard to completely avoid dining out, especially when celebrating birthdays, marriages, promotions, etc.

Because it's so common to use food as a tool for celebration rather than energy, it's nearly impossible not to get invited out to dinner to commemorate something important for somebody. If you can come up with a valid reason to decline an invite, then by all means do so, but you have to say yes sometimes.

When that time comes, show up to the venue prepared. If you can, pull the menu up online and make a healthy choice prior to your arrival. If you want to eat something that maybe doesn't fit into our guidelines, then scale back your calories during the rest of the day. Do NOT skip meals, just make them smaller. If you can, work out more intensely that morning.

Many restaurants now have light menu options, and list the calorie and fat content right on the menu. If you know you are going to be at one of those restaurants, your decision should be easy. If you're not sure, then refer to the paragraph above. Nearly all chain restaurants have their nutrition information online, if not on the menu.

You can have an appetizer, dessert or adult beverage, but rarely can you have all three without going over your calorie budget. Decide ahead of time which one you'd like the most.

Be prepared for peer pressure. Some of your less active friends may try to talk you into sharing a big greasy plate of chili cheese fries or mozzarella sticks, along with drinks and dessert. They may poke fun at you if you order a grilled chicken salad and pass on the appetizer. Don't let them get under your skin. Make the decision before you even go out that you won't be swayed from your path of dietary excellence. They can talk trash if they want to, but YOU are the one running marathons. What have THEY done lately? Remember, you are the one who determines what goes into your body.

Ask the waiter how your food is prepared. If it's deep fried and breaded, ask if you can have it baked or grilled. If something's sautéed in butter ask that it be sautéed in broth instead. Or, just choose another item. You can also ask that half of your meal be put in a doggy bag before they bring your plate. This way, you can keep the calorie count low and still enjoy something that doesn't fit into your every day eating plan. Just make sure you get right back on the track the following day. Don't allow a night of dining out to undo all of your hard work.

Bonus: Smoothies

Smoothies are an excellent way to stuff a bunch of nutrients into one glass. They taste great and are energizing before a run, and refreshing after one. When done right, they can even be used as a meal replacement.

Below are some smoothie recipes that are chock-full of the components you need to energize your running regimen. You may never touch another fatty cake again.

Before Running

Prior to running, you want a smoothie loaded with carbs to keep you energized during your workout. You don't want to fill it with too many protein laden items, simply because you may feel too full during the run. Below are some good recipes to fuel up prior to hitting the road. Measurements are not used, as it's best to mix smoothies to taste. You won't reap the benefits of a smoothie if you don't like the taste and end up not drinking it. Ginger and lemon juice goes a *long* way in giving a good flavor to smoothies that may otherwise not taste great.

The Incredible Hulk
-Kale leaves
-Romaine lettuce

-Mango Chunks
-Pineapple Chunks
-Fresh Ginger

Blend ingredients with ice until desired consistency is reached. Drink and go. Don't worry, it tastes great despite the fact that it's green. Not only does this smoothie taste great, but it's full of carbohydrates for energy and antioxidants for health.

The Green Meanie
-Kale
-Cucumber Chunks
-Celery Chunks
-Lemon Juice
-Pear Chunks
-Fresh Ginger

Toss everything in a blender with some ice until you have the thickness you want. Like the Hulk, this smoothie tastes better than it looks, thanks to the lemon and ginger. The cucumber and celery are full of water, helping you hydrate, while the pear provides your carbs. Kale is a super food full of essential nutrients.

Banana-Berry Bliss
-Strawberries
-Blackberries
-Raspberries
-Banana
-Splash of coconut water

Blend with ice until your smoothie is, well, smooth. Drink and run. The banana has potassium to help ward of muscle spasms. The berries have high water content for hydration and the coconut milk is a natural source of electrolytes. This is a great smoothie before long distance run.

It's a date
-Bananas
-Pitted fresh dates
-Flaxseed
-Peanut or almond butter
-Honey
-Almond milk

Blend with ice to create your preferred consistency. Drink and go. The almond milk and butter provide protein without making you feel too full. Bananas help prevent those annoying muscle spasms. Dates contain potassium as well, along with a long list of other health nutrients such as iron, calcium and vitamin B-6. Flaxseed is a good source of healthy Omega-3 fatty acids, which help prevent heart disease and some cancers.

All of the smoothies we've given you are great for more than just running. They all deliver a plethora of health benefits to undo the damage those fatty cakes may have caused. On a non-run day, these smoothies can still be consumed as part of breakfast, if you wish.

After Running

There are two ways to replenish your body after a run. You can use the "before" smoothie recipes and add a protein source to them (or have a hardboiled egg on the side) for muscle recovery, or you can use one of the recipes below. The recipes below will help replace the carbohydrates burned during your run, and they taste amazing. Don't pick up a donut or bacon-cheese burger following a run, thinking it's ok because you just ran. To stay healthy and energized, diet and exercise need to work together.

Espresso Excellence
-Vanilla flavored non-fat yogurt
-Instant coffee grounds
-Plain almond milk
-Hazelnut or almond extract (optional)
-Ice

Blend until smooth and enjoy a tasty recovery. This smoothie is great for the runner that loves caffeine. What's awesome about caffeine is that when used correctly (that means not drinking coffee and energy drinks throughout the day to replace sleep or healthy food) it may help you recover faster. This smoothie gives you your caffeine fix, along with that protein and carb combo that we keep preaching to you. Eat this smoothie with a side of fruit though, so you don't miss out on the nutrients.

Bring on the Berries
-Plain Greek Yogurt

-Frozen mixed berries (your choice)
-Flax seed
-Almond milk
-Ice
-Honey

Place ingredients in your blender and blend until you get the right thickness. This smoothie doesn't just help you recover and replenish your carbs, but it delivers a huge dose of disease fighting antioxidants. For the strongest antioxidant effect, choose a berry mix that has blueberries.

Cherry-Almond Awesomeness
-Pitted Cherries
-Almond Milk
-Almond Extract
-Vanilla Flavored, fat free yogurt
-Ice

Blend ingredients until smooth. Enjoy. The almond milk and yogurt provide protein and carbs, while the cherries give even more carbohydrates and some dietary fiber. This sweet treat is perfect for recovering after a distance run.

Tropical Get-A-Way
-Mango Chunks
-Pineapple chunks
-Banana slices
-Coconut Milk
-Low Fat Milk
-Vanilla Extract

-Ice

Puree ingredients until the desired consistency is reached. Enjoy the recovery benefits of the protein and carbohydrates in the milk, the antioxidants in the fruits and the electrolytes in the coconut milk.

Chocolate Banana Blast
-Banana
-Fat Free vanilla frozen yogurt
-Unsweetened Cocoa Powder
-Vanilla Extract
-Low-fat milk, soymilk or almond milk

Remember how we mentioned chocolate milk as being an excellent recovery drink? Well here's chocolate milk, supersized! Blend ingredients together to get a milkshake-like texture and enjoy. In addition to the protein and carbohydrate benefits of the milk and yogurt, you'll reap the potassium replacement benefits of the banana. All this, plus great taste makes this an outstanding choice for recovery!

These are just a small sampling of the types of smoothies you can make. For more recipes, see the Resource section at the end of this guide for an excellent book, Smoothies For Runners to get many more delicious smoothie recipes.

Supplements: Do You REALLY Need Them?

The short answer to this question is NO. You don't need supplements. In case you didn't notice, none of our smoothie recipes or meal ideas included protein powders, or other seemingly magical formulas for weight loss or muscle gain.

Scientists and dieticians haven't figured out why, but nutrients are best absorbed by the body when the body gets them in the form of FOOD. This is strictly speculation, but perhaps the body doesn't recognize powders, pills and potions as actual food, because THEY AREN'T.

Another problem with supplements? They aren't regulated by the Food and Drug Administration (FDA). Basically just about anyone can create a supplement and market it. You might be buying supplements created by your average Joe who thinks that what he sees on television qualifies him to give dietary advice. Remember the whole ephedrine fiasco? Do you really want to risk it?

 If you are eating right to begin with, supplements are not even necessary. Besides, most people think that supplements are more than just that, supplements. You can't eat doughnuts and fried chicken all day, then throw some whey-protein in your overly-sugary drink and expect to get positive results. Your best choice is to follow our dieting guidelines and make healthy eating and active living a lifestyle choice, not temporary periods of time in which you just want to lose weight or get stronger. Keeping up with a healthy lifestyle is easier than catching up every time you fall off the wagon.

There are two exceptions to this rule though. Multi-vitamins and fish oil pills can help round out your diet without the health risks that may be associated with other supplements. Many people, despite their best efforts don't get enough calcium or vitamin D. This is especially true for women. You can get an extra boost of both from a daily multi-vitamin. The Omega-3 fatty acid in fish oil is absorbed just as well in pill form as it is in food form. If you don't care for fish, or don't care to pay the sometimes outrageous prices of it, you can get similar health benefits from a daily fish oil pill.

If you choose to ignore our advice and stock up on pills, powders and potions regardless, fine. Don't say we didn't warn you. At least consult with your physician first, and get clearance from him or her. Make sure you always let your doctor know what supplements you are taking during your visits, so he or she can properly evaluate you and your health.

Sports Drinks: Drink Up or Forget About Them?

The answer to this question really depends on how much you actually run and work out in general. The more you exercise, the more sense it makes to drink sports drinks. They are chock full of calories, so you need to be extremely active for them to be metabolized efficiently.

Sports drinks help to replace electrolytes after an intense sweat session, which is good for your recovery, but electrolytes can also be found in less sugary sources such as coconut water and a variety of foods. Electrolyte replacement is extremely important, but your body shouldn't rely on overly-sweet sports drinks to get them.

Our ancestors didn't need sports drinks to replace their electrolytes and neither do you! Spoiler Alert: You'll see references to our ancestors more than once.

Besides, those drinks don't have all of the electrolytes you need. They typically provide two or three. There are six electrolytes that your body needs. These electrically-charged ions aid your body in balancing your blood chemicals and moving your muscles. The six electrolytes your body needs are sodium, magnesium, phosphate, potassium, calcium, and chloride. Some of these should sound familiar to you. We have mentioned potassium and calcium quite a few times already. Chloride is found in salt. Typically, your food has enough salt and you don't need to add any to your diet to get the chloride you need. Sodium is provided in salt as well. Does the term "sodium chloride" ring a bell? The whole grains we've been preaching all along will supply you with a magnesium boost, and phosphorus is found in eggs, lean meats and nuts.

So basically, if you are eating per our recommendations, sports drinks are not very necessary.

If you don't like the taste of sports drinks, or if the calorie content scares you, don't worry. You will not dehydrate and suffer a sports-related injury simply because you don't consume sports drinks. They are not the only means of recovery.

We are not going to say that you should eliminate your sports drinks, as many love the taste of them, and they are not the worst thing you can consume, but we aren't going to say they are essential to your diet either. Many of the commercials will have you believing that they are the only thing on the planet that can replace your electrolytes. This is simply not true. There are other ways to replenish what's lost from a work out.

Use your own discretion on this, but don't get carried away. You can consume too many calories and not enough nutrients if you rely on sports drinks.

Drink judiciously.

Meal Replacement Bars/Energy Bars: Are they as good as they seem?

Advertisements make you think protein bars are they key to your total body transformation. They'll have you thinking wrong. While they ARE better than fatty cakes and deep fried disaster, they aren't the secret to your dietary or running success.

In fact the "secret" to your success is actually no secret at all. Expend more calories than you consume, get enough sleep, maintain a good balance of cardio and strength training and you'll see changes in your body before you know it. If there was a way to get fit overnight, don't you think everyone would be ripped and bikini ready all the time? Well, not everyone is, because it's NOT easy and there's no magical concoction to eliminate the work involved in fitness.

Let's think about this for a minute. Our hunting and gathering ancestors did **much** more strenuous work than we do today. (Can you take down an elephant with just a spear and a prayer? We thought not). And they survived just fine without the packaged, processed and tasteless protein bars. Granted, they didn't live as long, but that was more because of a lack of medical aid and because shelters weren't so advanced, so the elements got to them faster. Their diet alone wasn't responsible for their early demise. In fact, with our medical technology, if we ate like our ancestors we'd probably live to be 150. Their food was one-hundred percent organic and unprocessed.

Since these bars are often low fat, they end up being high in sugar. Worse, some have no fat OR sugar, which means some sort of chemical blend with words you can't pronounce, is responsible for the bars' flavor (or lack thereof). That doesn't even sound like a good time does it?

Some of these bars are nothing but baked lumps of refined sugars and unhealthy fats. Throughout this book we mention the evils of both of those. They are no less evil in a "health bar" than they are in any other food.

Besides, we've already mentioned that food should look as close to its original form as possible. Can you think of any food on this earth that looks like a small rectangular bar naturally? Please, let us know if you do. You don't though, because food just doesn't grow like that. There is still a level processing involved to create these protein bars and meal replacements. We don't like processed food and think it should be avoided to the fullest extent possible.

If you are on the go and need a quick meal, some of these bars are alright, but by no means should you depend on them for your nutrition. We would rather you consume meal replacement bars than those fatty cakes, but there are better options to fuel your running efforts.

Don't get caught up in believing that these bars are the key to your stellar performance or that they will take you from an intermediate athlete to an Olympian. If this were true, we'd have a lot more Olympians!

If you must indulge in one of these, for convenience purposes look for ones that are organic, made from whole grains and low in fat. Never buy or eat anything that has trans-fat in it.

Another option: organic trail mix. It's always nice to be able to actually SEE what you are eating, rather than reading about it on a label. Proceed with caution here though. While trail mix does provide a very good mix of healthy fats and proteins, some contain sugars and nearly all of them are high in calories because of the nuts. If you are counting calories bear in mind that trail mix might break your calorie budget.

The Right Way to Hydrate

Of course runners need to drink water. In fact, even lazy couch potatoes need it, but runners need more. When you run, you sweat. When you sweat, you lose water. Since the human body is composed of so much water, it's important to replenish it after a major sweat session. None of your organs can function without it.

Hydration isn't just to replace the water you sweat out during a workout. Hydration keeps your body cool and regulates your core temperature. Think of your body as an engine. If your radiator has ever run out of water, you know what a disaster that is. Granted, your body won't blow up like your engine without water, but your systems will shut down and turn into a medical emergency. Besides saving your life, proper hydration is linked to a clearer complexion and more energy. So….Hydrate!

This all seems obvious right? Ok, well do you know how to hydrate according to the weather? You might think you need more water when it's hot out, but depending on how you dress during your workout, this may not be true.

More heat injuries occur in the winter months than warmer seasons, because when you bundle up in layers, your body heats up faster. Because of the cold, you may not notice it right away, then all of a sudden… BAM, you're suffering from heat exhaustion, or worse.

To avoid becoming a very preventable medical emergency, HYDRATE, HYDRATE, HYDRATE!

Since we've covered sports drinks already, we won't go down that road, but we will explain how to stay hydrated with proper food and water.

First off, you have likely been told your entire life that you need eight glasses of water per day, every day, for the rest of your life. This is true, but it's also not true. Let us explain. The amount of water in eight 8oz glasses of water IS how much you need, but it doesn't all have to come from water in a glass. Check the water content of your food.

Many items in your refrigerator likely have a high water content and will hydrate you just as effectively as water, and will *also* provide you with some other nutritional benefits that water doesn't offer. Foods high in water include:

-cucumbers
-celery
-watermelon
-cantaloupe
-strawberries
-oranges
-apples
-lettuce
-broccoli

-milk
-honeydew
-mangos

Any of these options, and many, many more will supply you with more than just water. You'll also get your electrolyte fill (as discussed previously) and the vitamins, minerals and antioxidants found in all of them. Not that water is BAD for you. Please don't stop drinking it! However, there are hydration options that offer more of a nutrition benefit than water alone.

We're not saying you can give water up. Depending on the intensity of your workouts, you may need to stick to your eight glasses a day *and* increase the amounts of water rich foods you consume. You may also need to adjust your intake depending on the weather. In summer months, if you spend a lot of time outdoors, you may lose water without even working out.

In winter months, when cold and flu viruses are running rampant, you may want to "eat your water" more than you do in the summer, because most of your options contain disease fighting antioxidants and immune boosting vitamin C. You can't necessarily avoid every virus in your home or office, but you can hopefully ward off a few of them by eating right.

How much water you need depends on how much sweat you lose from a workout. An easy way to monitor your fluid losses is to simply look at your urine.

If it looks clear or very pale yellow, you are sufficiently hydrated. If it looks radioactive yellow and/or smells strong, it's time to hydrate. You can't really measure the exact amount of water you've lost but you can know when it's time to replace it. Don't wait until your urine is bright though, to hydrate (Note: Many multi-vitamins can make your urine yellow or bright yellow). Drink water and eat water-heavy foods throughout the day so that you never reach the point at which your urine looks and smells disgusting.

Thirst is a sign of mild hydration. You should drink and eat enough to prevent thirst from setting in to begin with, which will in turn prevent you from having to see neon yellow urine in the bathroom.

Not only can dehydration become life-threatening if it's not taken care of, but it can degrade your athletic performance. No one wants to pass out on the track.

With that being said, follow our hydration tips and you'll perform at your best while avoiding the drama of an ER visit.

Time to Get Juiced... or Not

Like sports drinks and meal replacement bars, manufacturers will try to convince you that so long as you drink their "fortified, enriched" drinks that you'll live to be 100 and run like the wind.

As nice as this sounds, it is of course, untrue. Now, we aren't saying orange juice with calcium is bad for you, or that milk with vitamin D is bad. It's rarely a bad idea to give your body extra nutrients when possible. However, you do not *need* to consume these juices.

If you are following our guidance and eating mindfully, you'll likely be taking in enough of everything anyway. The only time we'd tell you that fortified juices are really a necessity is if you have a condition that makes you deficient in an essential vitamin or mineral. For example, if you have anemia or other iron deficiency, then drinking some iron fortified juice can only help you out.

What's even better than enriched juices? Making your own. If you put the right items in your juice extractor, you'll get a huge dose of vitamins and minerals and add to your water quota for the day as well. Read below for our best juicing recipes.

Melon-Berrylicious
 -Strawberries
 -Watermelon
 -Peaches
 -Mango

Add ingredients to your juicer and extract as much as you can. Drink over ice or refrigerate before serving. Bear in mind, the juices you make at home will be somewhat thicker than those you buy in the store, because they have no added water. If the consistency bothers you, feel free to add some water. The recipe above can also be made into a smoothie, but some of the ones that follow wouldn't be very tasty as smoothies. Use your own discretion.

Ever Green
 -Kale
 -Cucumber
 -Spinach
 -Kale
 -Celery Stalks
 -Lemon Juice
 -Ginger

This is one of the recipes that we don't recommend as a smoothie. We do have a few green smoothies, but this isn't one of them. Put everything in your extractor and juice away. Enjoy.

Orange Carrot

-Oranges

-Carrots

Yes, that's all you need for this one. This also won't make a very tasty smoothie. It does however, make a great juice. The carrot tames the tang of the oranges and the oranges give it just enough sweetness. Oranges deliver a good amount of water and vitamin C and the carrots have vitamin A. Oh, and your mom was right. Carrots can help your eyesight!

Awesome Cran-Apple

-Red apples

-Cranberries

-Grapes (any color)

Place items in you juicer and extract until there's nothing left to extract. Drink up. This water rich combo tastes great and is a good way to hydrate if you're bored with water.

Pina Colada

-Pineapple

-Coconut water

Juice the pineapple only. Add the coconut water and embark on your tropical getaway. Hold the Captain Morgan's. Rum has tons of calories.

Bloody Mary

-Tomatoes

-Cucumbers

-Celery
-Parsley
-Spinach

Juice it up and enjoy with a splash of hot sauce if you need some extra flavor. Pass on the vodka. It dehydrates you.

All of these recipes can be used in place of fortified drinks and provide most of the same benefits. Most of them taste better and they don't contain any craziness such refined sugar or high-fructose corn syrup, like many store bought options do. Also, you'll know exactly what is in your drinks, saving you the hassle of trying to pronounce the things found on commercial ingredient lists and looking them up online.

Make enough to fill up a pitcher at the beginning of each week to save you some time. Now, you have a ready-made recovery drink to enjoy with all of our meals and snacks.

If you really feel the need to drink juices with all the extra bells and whistles, opt for organic or all natural choices to avoid refined sugars and high fructose corn syrup. Fruit is usually sweet on its own. There's no need to add sugars to it most of the time.

Note that there was no point at which we suggested a juice fast. Runners can **not** afford to skip out on solid foods. Juicing will deprive you of essentials such as proteins and calcium, so it's best to have these juices with or between meals, not INSTEAD of meals. Besides, people get mean and moody when they're hungry. Don't be that guy. He's not attractive.

We don't subscribe to the philosophy of juice cleansing. If you eat right you'll undo any damage you've done with bad food choices. There's no need to starve yourself to reset your system.

Catch Some Z's

Ok, so it's not directly related to food, but sleep is essential. In our busy lives, we often forget this one simple fact. While many say eight hours is the magic number, you may need more, or less, depending on your age, activity level and your individual needs.

Sleep is your body's opportunity to rest and repair itself from the damages done throughout the day. While sleeping, your systems are basically reset and ready to perform the following day, provided you get enough sleep. Enough GOOD sleep that is.

To determine how much you need, try to wake up without an alarm clock for a few days, after going to sleep at the same time every night. This will clue you in to your circadian rhythms and help you determine how many hours of sleep are right for you.

Sleep deprivation can cause a range of issues from weight gain to decreased memory. If you've ever embarked on a distance run after staying up too late and getting up to early, you know exactly how important sleep is. It's nearly impossible to perform at your peak when you're tired and groggy from late nights.

The quality of your sleep is just as important how many hours of sleep you log each night. The type of sleep you need to effectively restore yourself is the deep sleep that you enter during rapid eye movement (REM) sleep. This is the sleep in which your subconscious is in charge and your conscious body and mind get to relax and chill out.

Improve the quality of your sleep by eliminating distractions and having a bedtime routine. Those readers who have children might know what I'm talking about. Routine is just as important for adults though. Distractions such as lights from your electronics and noise from your television can lessen the quality of your sleep. So can having a bad mattress, and *not* having a sleeping routine. Try to go to bed and wake up at the same time every day, even on weekends. We know it's easier said than done, but try it anyway.

Several hours before bedtime, avoid caffeine, alcohol, the television and the computer. Caffeine is of course a stimulant that will keep you awaken when you need to sleep. Alcohol, while it may make you feel sleepy, it won't keep you asleep through the night. When you try to sleep under the influence, you will likely find yourself waking up in the middle of the night, or staying asleep but having crazy psychedelic dreams that compromise your sleep quality. TV, computers and other electronics stimulate your brain and make it hard to turn it off when you're trying to rack out.

Check the temperature of your house. While you're sleeping, your core temperature drops slightly. Setting your thermostat a few degrees lower about 30 minutes before you want to fall asleep, signals your body that it's time to slow down.

Don't work out prior to going to bed either. As most athletes know, exercise gives you a burst of energy and stimulates your mind. It can take up to two hours to come down from your runner's high. If you exercise late in the day, try to finish at least three hours prior to your scheduled bedtime.

Find a relaxing activity to do before you go to bed. Try taking a warm bath, which will help your body temperature drop. As mentioned, this will help your body know that it's time to sleep. Reading, writing and meditating are good options as well. If you're having trouble falling asleep, try tricking your mind. Try to keep your eyes open as long as possible and you just might drift off.

Sometimes worries such as finances, relationship issues, car repairs, social obligations and the like can keep you awake. If something like this is keeping you up, try writing a list of what's bothering you right before you go to bed. This helps you verbalize what's bothering you and makes problems seem more manageable.

In extreme cases of sleep deprivation you may need to see a doctor who can prescribe a sedative or a therapist that will help you better deal with your issues. You may be suffering from Post Traumatic Stress Disorder or anxiety problems that we are not equipped to diagnose and treat. If you go more than three nights a week without adequate sleep, you should get an expert opinion.

What to Avoid

Being a runner is hard work right? Right. So don't undo all of your hard work by over-indulging in foods and drinks that will cancel out everything you've worked so diligently for. This is especially important if you have been working to lose weight and get lean and healthy. It's much easier to maintain your healthy weight and a level of fitness than it is to get to those levels from a not-so-healthy state of being.

Being healthy isn't all about your weight, although that's part of it. Staying fit and active can reduce your risk of heart disease, cancer and common ailments such as colds or the flu. You can also stave off diabetes if you eat right and stay active.

What follows is a list of the things you should avoid as much as possible, as they will reverse the effects of your healthy and active lifestyle.

Alcohol

We aren't saying you can never drink again, but we are saying to do so *in moderation*. Most drinks are full of sugars and calories. Also, working out is never a good time when you're hung over. Alcohol dehydrates you. We've explained how bad dehydration is for your health and performance, so it's rather silly to purposefully engage in an activity that puts you at risk.

You may have heard that having three ounces of red wine each night after dinner has been shown to help prevent cancer and heart disease, but please don't think you can have that one glass each night, skip workouts and eat crap and still get the effects. Red wine is a side dish of a healthy diet, *not* an entrée. Oh, and don't think you can abstain from alcohol all week and drink an entire bottle of red wine on the weekend and get the same benefits. You'll just get a wine headache and hangover.

If you are at a social gathering and really feel as though you want to imbibe, look for low calorie drinks such as light beer or tequila and lime. Limit yourself to two drinks and cut back the calories in one of your meals on the days you know alcohols will be involved.

Refined Sugars and Carbohydrates

We've mentioned this over and over again, but we feel as though we should bring it up again. Studies have shown that people who avoid refined starches and sugars have a lower body mass than those who don't. They tend to live longer and healthier lives. Remember, the simple carbohydrates found naturally in fruits and vegetables are fine. It's those grains that are processed and stripped of everything good for you that you need to be aware of, and avoid. Things like candy, white bread, cakes, cookies and white flour pastas are all examples of the carbs you want to avoid. The sugars found in many of these can actually become addictive, causing you to want more and more, which of course makes you gain more and more. To avoid the addiction, don't over-indulge. You know what else has refined sugars? Fatty cakes. Leave them alone! Ice cream has one of the highest fat and sugar content of almost any food. Try to avoid ice cream at all costs. Reduced fat or "low cal" ice creams will be filled with chemicals and artificial sweeteners, another toxic mix.

Smoking

Besides being disgusting, smoking puts you at risk for a plethora of health problems. Long term smokers are all but guaranteed to contract lung cancer at some point in their lives. Smokers are also prone to stomach cancer, oral cancer, kidney cancer, cervical cancer, leukemia, pancreatic cancer and esophageal cancer. That's the short list of problems caused by smoking. You shouldn't be surprised. You've been told about the evils of tobacco since grade school. Yet, many people still choose to pick up the habit.

Tobacco is toxic and so full poisons that can damage basically every part of your body. Come on people! Tobacco has arsenic in it for goodness sake! You would never sprinkle that on in your food or drinks, so why on earth would you smoke it? The reasons are beyond us.

Smoking also degrades your performances. Because one of the primary organs affected by cigarette smoke is the lungs, many smokers have respiratory issues. Runners need to be able to breathe properly to get life-giving oxygen to their muscles and organs.

If you're not a smoker, keep up the good work. If you ARE, please seriously consider dropping the habit. No good can come from tobacco use. The same dangers apply to dip and chew. Just say NO.

Protein powder/Creatin Powder/Other non-FDA regulated powders

First of all, if you're reading this you're a runner. You're not a body builder. So, all those extras are just not necessary to your fitness. We've covered it before, but decided to mention it again. Don't pay for things that the FDA doesn't regulate. When you use these additives, you're putting yourself at risk for whatever health problem they can cause. Do you really want to be the guy whose heart exploded from some manufactured supplements that hadn't been adequately researched? You don't need them anyway, if you're eating right. We'll refer back to the example we used about our ancestors. They didn't need any of this stuff and neither do you.

If you're going to be stubborn and use it anyway, proceed with caution and notify your doctor beforehand.

Counting Calories: Do You Really Need To?

Well, yes you do. But, no, you don't. See, the calories in/calories out formula isn't necessary if you're healthy, at your desired weight and pleased with how you look. If what you're doing now isn't broke, don't fix it.

However, if you are trying to lose a few pounds, you may benefit from counting your calories for at least a couple of weeks. Often, we eat much more than we're aware of. Having a small spoonful of cake batter won't make you blow up like a balloon. The problem with this is, if you keep having those small spoonfuls, things start to add up faster than you may like.

Another issue: people tend to over-estimate the number of calories they are expending and underestimate what they are consuming. Too often, people take what the exercise machine says to heart. The number of calories the machine says you're burning is typically grossly inaccurate. About ninety percent of the time, these machines will give a higher number than the truth, giving you a false sense of security.

To ensure you're on the right track to weight loss, counting calories is a necessity, at least until you are more aware of the calories you are taking in versus the calories you are expending. Many smartphones now have free weight loss applications such as Lose-it and MyFitnessPal. Such apps allow you to record your food and exercise on a daily basis and they calculate your net calories for you. So long as you're under on most days, you're doing all the right things to lose the weight.

If you can't get these apps on your phone, or prefer to do things the old fashioned way, consider keeping a food journal. Record every bite to gain insight into your eating habits. Do you eat salty fatty foods when you're stressed? Do you eat when you're bored? Recognizing such behaviors can help you modify or eliminate them. Becoming mindful of what you're eating, when you're eating it my help you stop that ice cream and potato chip binge before you start.

Once you have a firm grasp on your calories in/calories out ratio, you can ease up on calorie counting. Doing it for a couple of weeks will help you identify what works for you and what doesn't.

If you're working out regularly and eating a diet that follows our guidelines, counting calories may not even be a necessity, but if other methods of weight loss haven't worked for you, then some calorie math may be the key to your success.

So Now You Know

If you have been trying to improve your running performance, a shift in your diet might be just what you need. The right balance in your diet might be exactly what you need to take your running game to the next level.

Remember the basics, sixty percent **unrefined** carbohydrates, thirty percent protein and fill in the rest with healthy fats that don't come from animal sources. Stick to this balance as closely as you can, get enough sleep and stay hydrated. Following these simple, but often unheeded guidelines will get you on track to your personal best.

We've armed you with the knowledge you need to fuel yourself for top performance, so we don't want to hear any more excuses from you! Put down the junk food and hit the track!

Recommended Resources

RunnersDepot.org – A full line of all things running

Smoothies For Runners – Excellent book for runners and smoothie lovers alike!

Also by J. M. Parker

The Ultimate Running Guide: How To Train For a 5K, 10K, Half-Marathon or Full Marathon (Kindle edition)

The Ultimate Running Guide (Paperback edition)

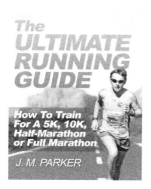

Made in the USA
Coppell, TX
06 November 2024

39743223R20046